Morning pregnancy workout

Energizing Exercises for a Healthy Pregnancy Start

Dr. Betty C. Redding

Table of contents

Introduction

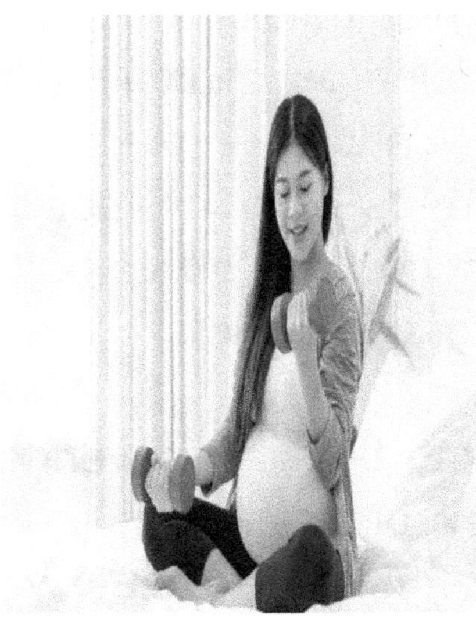

When it comes to maintaining shape during pregnancy, exercise is a requirement. Expectant women may preserve their physical condition while also promoting a healthy pregnancy with a suitable workout plan.

Dr. Betty C. Redding's book Morning Pregnancy Workout gives a full introduction to prenatal exercise with simple, safe, and effective activities.

This book, which relies on several subjects, including psychology and cognitive science, presents expecting parents with an easily accessible way to keep active both during and after pregnancy.

Betty starts the book by covering the physiology of pregnancy and the risks connected with excessive physical exertion.

She presents a full discussion of how to assess and alter intensity levels depending on the pregnancy stage, with an emphasis on anaerobic exercise.

Betty also emphasizes the psychological benefits of physical exercise during this time, emphasizing stress reduction and metabolic improvement.

Moving on to the exercises themselves, Betty provides a range of regimens aimed to increase flexibility, strength, balance, and coordination.

Each exercise is offered in basic steps, with images and diagrams illustrating suitable techniques. Betty also advises having appropriate aims and avoiding overtraining, supporting expectant women in nourishing not only the body but also the mentality.

Morning Pregnancy Workout is a fantastic resource for any pregnant lady striving to maintain shape. Dr. Betty' grasp of the psychological and physiological components of pregnant exercise creates a clear and complete regimen that is easy to follow.

 This book will surely improve both the body and emotions of any pregnant lady.

Chapter 1

The Advantages of Morning Exercises During Pregnancy

Pregnancy morning workouts may be a superb approach for expecting mums to be healthy and active throughout their pregnancy.

Working activities in the morning

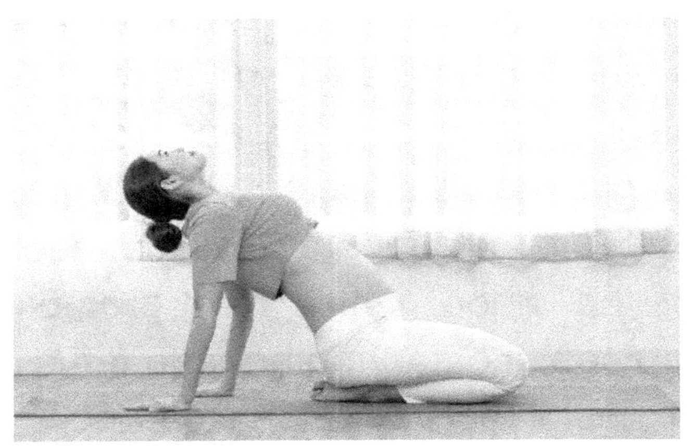

may deliver various benefits,

including better cardiovascular health, mood and energy, and sleep quality.

Expectant women may be better informed about the advantages of morning activities throughout their pregnancy by knowing the scientific facts that support these claims.

Improved cardiovascular health is one of the most significant benefits of morning activities during pregnancy. Morning exercise has been demonstrated in studies to have a beneficial influence on the cardiovascular system, leading to better circulation and oxygenation of the blood, which may promote the health of the mother and fetus.

Regular activity during pregnancy may also aid to lessen the chance of gestational diabetes, which may be dangerous for both the mother and the baby.

Cardiovascular exercise helps boost metabolism and body composition during pregnancy, which is good for overall health.

Improved mood and energy levels are another advantage of early activities during pregnancy.

Regular exercise may enhance the synthesis of the "feel-good" neurotransmitters serotonin and dopamine, helping a pregnant woman feel more joyful and energetic.

Improved mood and energy levels may be especially useful for pregnant women who are weary or depressed, both of which may have a major effect on the mother's overall wellness.

Morning activities may also improve sleep quality during pregnancy. Exercise may lessen the time it takes to fall asleep and promote more restful sleep for longer amounts of time.

A better night's sleep may be crucial for a pregnant woman, especially during the first and third trimesters when the mother is more likely to feel exhausted.

Morning activities during pregnancy give various benefits for both the mother and the baby. Exercise not only improves cardiovascular health, mood, energy levels, and sleep quality, but it also improves body composition and metabolism.

Expectant parents should discuss their fitness needs with their healthcare specialists and consider adopting morning activities as a good way to promote a healthy pregnancy.

Chapter 2

Exercises for Morning Pregnancy Workouts

Nothing beats strength training regimens that are specifically geared to the changing needs of the body for pregnant women wanting to maintain healthy and fit while expecting.

These exercises are meant to target particular muscles and/or body areas harmed by pregnancy, as well as to tone and condition the muscles.

Exercises for morning pregnancy workouts will offer extensive guidance on the ideal for morning pregnancy workouts.

Workouts should always be adjusted to the individual's level of physical fitness and experience; pregnant women should always consult with their doctor and/or a fitness trainer before commencing any sort of exercise.

It is vital to listen to one's body during a workout and only pursue things that one can safely perform.

When arranging a morning pregnancy workout, consider the following types of exercises:

Light cardiovascular activities, such as walking, jogging, or cycling, may assist to keep the body warm while also delivering important nutrient circulation throughout the system.

It is vital to keep the intensity low and moderate and to not exceed

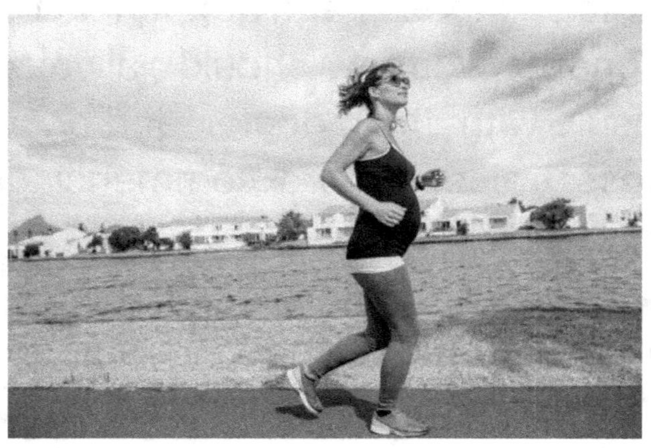

the intensity levels suggested by one's doctor.

Core Strengthening: Abdominal exercises such as pelvic tilts and plank variations aid the body sustain a growing baby.

Back stretches like the cobra and spinal twists may help prevent pregnancy-related postural irregularities and boost overall back health.

Bodyweight Exercises: Pregnancy is a good time to focus on bodyweight exercises such as squats, wall sits, and push-ups. These exercises may be done with small weights for a slightly more strenuous workout, or without weights for a reduced intensity.

Pilates and Yoga are both workout practices that promote core and body awareness. This is vital for pregnant women to measure stress on the body and determine suitable warm-ups and cool-downs.

Because it is low impact and helps to ease joint stress, swimming is one of the finest sorts of exercise for pregnant women. Swimming may deliver a terrific workout while providing a minimal threat of injury.

A morning pregnancy exercise may help you keep your overall physical fitness, prevent excessive weight gain, boost your sleep, and lessen your stress levels. It is crucial to remember not to push oneself too far and to maintain a sufficient degree of intensity.

A morning exercise routine, with suitable guidance and training, may be an essential component of a healthy pregnancy.

Chapter 3

Post-Workout Stretching and Cooling Down

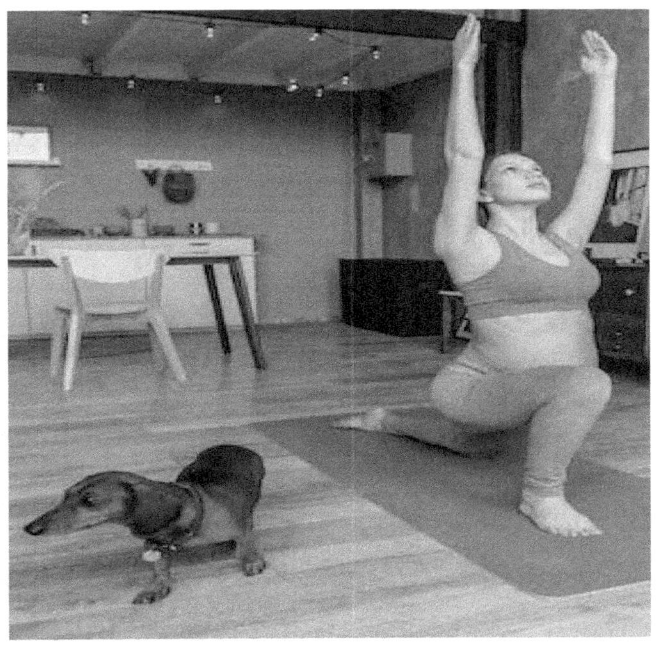

The third chapter of Morning Pregnancy training highlights the significance of stretching and cooling down after a training session.

These workouts aid to prevent muscle and joint aches and lessen the possibility of damage.

Stretching and cooling down may assist a pregnant woman's body, as well as exact advice for stretching and cooling down after a workout.

Stretching is excellent before and after exercise because it maintains muscles warm, relaxed, and supple, allowing for a greater range of motion and more effective movements. Stretching out tight and over-active muscles regularly is especially vital during pregnancy as it promotes flexibility and lowers the danger of damage.

Stretching after a workout helps to release stress and tension in the muscles, as well as promote circulation to freshly impacted areas.

Cooling down after exercise is also vital as it helps to slow the heart rate and minimizes the risk of dizziness or fainting.

When stretching after a pregnancy activity, it is essential to concentrate on the key muscle groups. Legs, core, back, and arms are examples.

Some of the greatest leg stretches involve stretching out the quadriceps, hamstrings, calves, and hips. Stretches like the cobra or bridge could be useful to the core. Half-cobra and cat-cow poses are wonderful for stretching out the back.

Stretching the chest and shoulder muscles could aid with arm soreness.

Cooling down after exercise is just as crucial as stretching the primary muscle groups.

Slower actions, such as modest and controlled walks or jogs, may aid restore the heart rate to its resting condition.

It may also entail modest leg and other muscular stretching. After exercise, cooling down requires hydrating and nourishing the body.

Stretching and cooling down are crucial during pregnancy, as well as guidelines for targeting primary muscle groups and cooling down after exercise.

Stretching out tight and overactive muscles, as well as cooling down after exertion, may aid keep the body and muscles safe and healthy throughout pregnancy.

Chapter 4

Working Out with Bodyweight Exercises During Pregnancy

The advantage of completing bodyweight workouts during pregnancy can be adapted to make a safe and effective workout for pregnant women.

While physical fitness is typically related to its outward effects, one of the most significant benefits of exercising during pregnancy is the inside adjustments it could produce.

Exercising during pregnancy enhances blood circulation and

subsequently oxygen levels, resulting in increased nutrient delivery to both the mother and her baby. It also assists in the regulation of stress and mood. The serene, quiet experience that a woman feels after exercising may ease anxiety and provide a sense

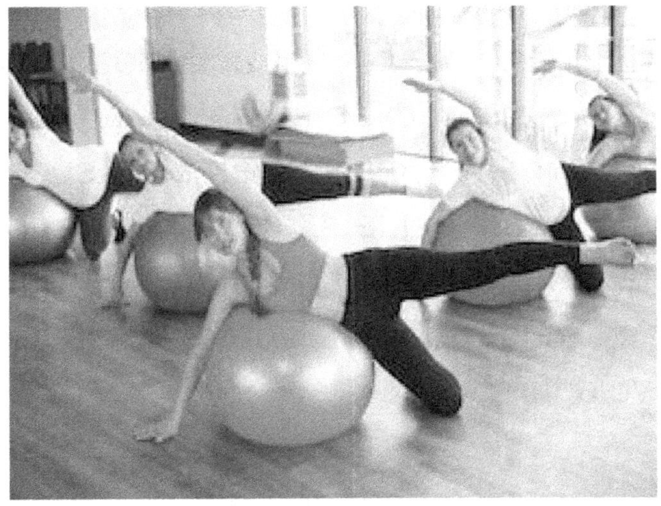

of emotional well-being.

Cardio is one of the most popular bodyweight exercises for pregnant women.
Walking at moderate-to-fast speeds encourages the heart to work harder while exerting less pressure on the joints.

Swimming and cycling are additional low-impact activities that enable the body to move freely.
Weight-bearing movements such as lunges, squats, crunches, and push-ups are also effective, but they must be done appropriately to avoid injury.

Warming up appropriately is one of the most crucial components of any pregnant workout. Without a warm-up, the danger of harm climbs considerably.

A fast 5-10 minute warm-up of modest, moderate jumps and active mobility exercises like arm and leg circles will aid prepare the body for safe activity.

Bodyweight exercises should be done at a conversational level; if they are too hard, the body will be unable to respond adequately.

Faster-paced exercises may be useful, but bear in mind that the aim is to boost the heart rate, not to exhaust the body.

Stretching and hydration should not be overlooked. Stretching after each exercise lowers soreness and promotes overall flexibility. Ample water drinking maintains the body hydrated and could help increase athletic performance.

Pregnant women may maintain physically and mentally healthy by undertaking bodyweight workouts.

Readers may guarantee that they begin or continue to conduct bodyweight exercises while pregnant safely and effectively by following the advice suggested in this chapter.

Chapter 5

Pregnancy Intensity Modification Guidelines

Exercising during pregnancy could be advantageous if you know how to control the intensity levels.

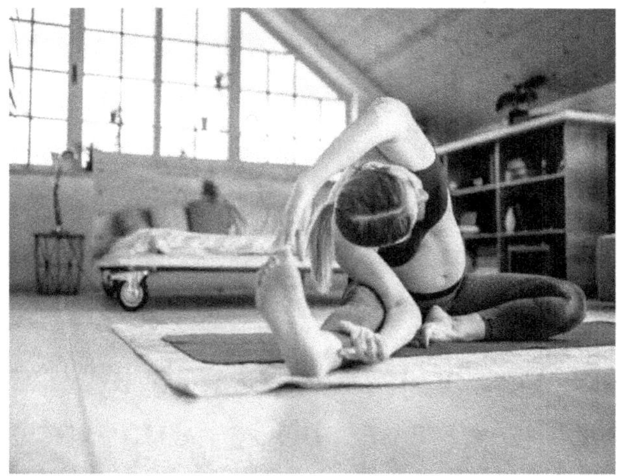

Understanding how to change intensity for your current fitness level, trimester, and training goals is crucial for a healthy and safe pregnancy.

It will not only keep you and your baby healthy, but it will also increase your overall well-being during the pregnancy.

When it comes to altering exercise intensity throughout pregnancy, each trimester requires you to change exercises depending on your current level of fitness and physical capabilities. Most pregnant women can continue with their typical exercises during the first trimester.

However, it is crucial to always be aware of your body and any probable pain or discomfort that can be a symptom of an overstressed body.

This means switching low-intensity exercises with ones that are suitable for your fitness level and current stage of pregnancy.

Light aerobic activities like walking, swimming, or cycling are normally safe for the first trimester, while hobbies like Pilates or yoga may help maintain strength and flexibility.

Your energy level is likely to rise in the second trimester, and your bump will start to develop.

Adjusting intensity throughout the second trimester will mean steadily upping the length and difficulty levels of your workouts during this period.

As your fitness level increases, you may start introducing moderate-intensity workouts like jogging and light weights. Any new interests should be treated with discretion.

During this trimester, it's crucial to be alert to indicators of weariness or discomfort and to respond immediately if you encounter pain or dizziness while exercising.

It's suggested to focus on low to moderate-intensity exercises that are suitable for your fitness level and the size of your bump during the third trimester.

Traditional exercises, such as walking or swimming, may be the most pleasurable and conveniently altered to meet your energy level and physical limits.

If you still want to practice weight lifting or other difficult workouts, be careful to adapt and apply alterations such as a narrower stance, lighter weights, and shorter sessions.

It is crucial to rest when required and to take frequent breaks if you are fatigued.

It is crucial to pay attention to your body and notice any symptoms of weariness or overexertion.

Staying vigilant and recognizing the crucial adjustments will aid you in modifying intensity and ensuring a safe and joyful training plan while pregnant.

Chapter 6

Common Obstacles to Pregnancy Exercise and Solutions

For many women, pregnancy may be   a

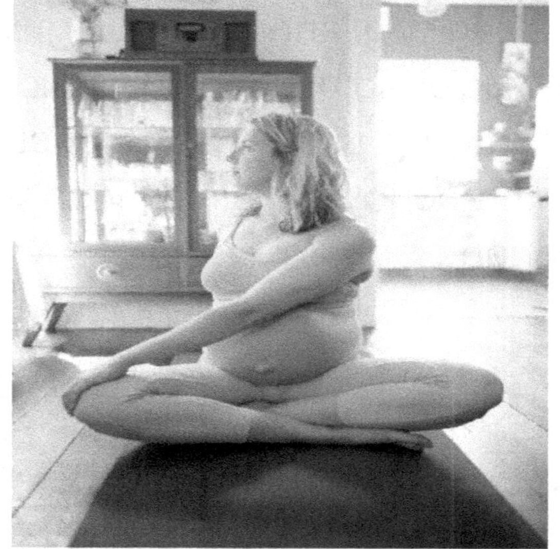

great, albeit stressful, moment in

their life. Many pregnant women may be anxious to begin a regular physical fitness program to maintain health and retain their mental well-being.

However, beginning or continuing a regular exercise plan during pregnancy can provide a variety of problems that may limit their development.

This chapter will look at some of these challenges and present advice for new and expecting women to remain on track with their workouts.

Exhaustion is one of the most typical issues that pregnant women experience. To different degrees, all pregnant women will endure weariness throughout their pregnancy, depending on the stage of pregnancy and the specific woman's overall health and well-being.

It is all too easy to fall prey to fatigue-driven arguments for not exercising or taking time off from your schedule.

It is vital to produce an appropriate speed and intensity to combat weariness and ensure that you continue to your training plan.

Begin gently and take breaks as necessary. Accepting low-impact physical activities like walking, swimming, and yoga may help you incorporate physical activity without placing undue pressure on your body.

It is common to feel fatigued during pregnancy, and it is crucial to listen to your body and rest when required.

Fear of injury and miscarriage is another usual fear that pregnant women may confront in their quest to be active.

Many people feel that physical activity during pregnancy is detrimental and increases a woman's probability of injury or miscarriage.

The reality is that frequent physical activity during pregnancy may enhance both the mother's and the baby's health. The objective is to pace each exercise session and moderate the intensity, frequency, and duration of workouts to prevent overexertion of the body.

Discuss your fitness aims with your doctor to verify that the training plan is safe for both you and your baby.

One of the most typical hurdles to going out throughout pregnancy is a **lack of excitement to be active**. It is typical to suffer emotional and mood changes while pregnant.

During this phase, it could be tough to find the energy and passion to prioritize exercise.

Establishing a routine is a vital step in building daily motivation and long-term habits. Schedule specific exercise times and seek to break down bigger objectives, such as weight loss or better endurance, into smaller, more realistic ambitions and short-term results.

Many women may realize that being a part of a group engaging in physical activity and goal-oriented training may provide extra encouragement and support, which may help sustain motivation throughout the pregnancy journey.

Obstacles to initiating and keeping an exercise plan during pregnancy abound for pregnant women.

Education and planning may help them anticipate and handle normal issues like weariness, injury worry, and difficulty remaining active.

Despite the obstacles that come with pregnancy, new moms may exercise safely and effectively to maintain physical, mental, and emotional well-being.

Chapter 7

Breathing Techniques for an Easier Workout

Learning suitable breathing practices is one of the most crucial parts of keeping a fantastic pregnancy fitness plan.

Physical exertion during pregnancy generally elevates respiration and heart rate, as well as feelings of worry.

As a consequence, expectant women must employ conscious breathing methods to ensure that they have adequate oxygen to meet their needs.

Paying attention to one's breathing may lower the intensity of the exercise and make it more acceptable for the pregnant woman.

Diaphragmatic breathing, sometimes known as abdominal or

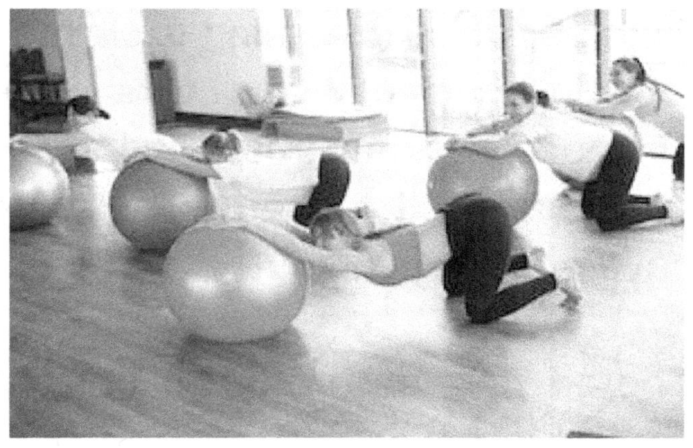

belly breathing, is the most frequent and effective breathing mode.

This technique requires the user to rest one hand on their abdomen while breathing deeply and slowly, causing their belly to rise and fall rather than their chest.

While doing so, the individual may envision their complete body rising with each inhale and then dropping with each exhale. Diaphragmatic breathing is claimed to help boost oxygen intake while also decreasing stress and pulse rate, making it a useful method to have during a workout.

The 4-7-8 method is another useful breathing technique. This strategy may be applied to boost lung capacity and calm the body.

This is performed by initially breathing for four seconds, holding their breath for seven seconds, and then exhaling for eight seconds.

This activity is believed to greatly calm the body, resulting in a sensation of tranquility and delivering increased stamina.

Abdominal lock breathing, in addition to diaphragmatic breathing and the 4-7-8 technique, may be advantageous, particularly during exercises that need core stability (such as planks or yoga poses).

This style of breathing is performed by inhaling slowly and deeply through the abdomen and then expelling abruptly. This technique instructs the user to create a double abdominal breath contraction while simultaneously pushing the abdomen or core outward.

This action not only improves stability during the exercise but also encourages deeper breathing. In addition to the kinds of breathing outlined above, it is vital to pay attention to the breath's rhythm.

This includes achieving the correct balance between intensity and number of breaths taken.

Pregnancy workouts must be correctly scheduled to ensure that breathing does not become too strained or hard.

Finding a regular and controlled breathing pattern may enable a pregnant woman to more easily manage the intensity of their activity while also supplying essential oxygen throughout the workout.

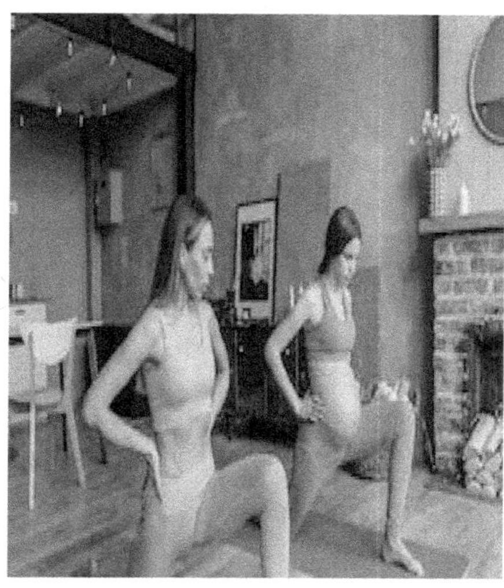

Cognitive breathing practices are just as crucial as physical exercise for an efficient pregnancy fitness plan.

Expectant mothers may ensure that their workouts are pleasant and that they have adequate oxygen by following the techniques indicated above, such as diaphragmatic breathing, the 4-7-8 method, and abdominal lock breathing.

Pregnancy workouts may be done and managed efficiently if these tips are followed.

Conclusion

Morning Pregnancy Workout is a pregnancy workout that has the potential to be highly useful to pregnant women.

The book highlights the necessity of a proper diet and exercise before, during, and after pregnancy, and encourages pregnant women to partake in moderate activity for their well-being.

Any potential dangers or risks related to exercise during pregnancy should be reviewed with a healthcare practitioner so that any exercise plan may be customized to the individual needs of each pregnant woman.

Pregnant women may be certain that with the correct adaptations, exercise may be a safe and effective strategy to maintain fit and strong throughout their pregnancy.